YOUR INTRODUCTION TO YOGA

Achieving greater mental health and body wellness

Written by M. J. Landon

Jikno Publishing©

Table of Contents

Table of Contents

Introduction

Are you new to Yoga? Do you feel scared about joining a Yoga class? Well, trust me, you are not alone. Getting started as a Yoga beginner can be seen as intimidating, but you can rest assured that you found a safe introduction in this book, you're in the right place. The fact that you have thought about starting Yoga classes and even went a step further to read this beginner's guide means that you belong here. You are qualified and ready for the leap of faith.

So many people think that yoga is for a certain class of people, skin color, body type, the rich or some preconceived notions like these. The truth is, yoga is for everyone, irrespective of what or who you think you are. The only difference is that people allow their thoughts to limit their willingness to take up yoga seriously.

One thing that you have to bear in mind is that with yoga, you can accomplish anything. You can clear your mind and do something awesome for yourself. When you make up your mind to start yoga classes, brace yourself, hold your head up and your shoulders high and walk into that class with lots of confidence. When you know that everyone is welcome to yoga and that you will be guided through practice, then you know that you are not alone!

Over the last several decades, yoga has gained so much popularity among people across the world. The truth is, so much research has gone into studying yoga and its benefits. While some people think of yoga as a fad, the truth is that results speak louder than words. I can personally vouch how amazing this form of exercise is and makes you feel about yourself.

You may be thinking "but what is yoga?" Well, if you ask this question to people, you will be amazed by the responses you get. To some, yoga is a way that makes their bodies feel good. To others, it is referred to as a spiritual practice, and to others, yoga is a lifestyle! However, regardless of how you define yoga, one thing's certain - this exercise will help you shape your life and discover both your conscious and unconscious habitual patterns.

It is important to acknowledge that yoga offers a foundation for you to build your life from the ground up. You can build good habits such as kindness, self-discipline, and self-inquiry which eventually contributes to your self-esteem and confidence. Indeed, yoga is the pathway to empowering your conscious decisions so that you can live a healthy and fuller life. This explains the true meaning of yoga, which is derived from the word *"yuj"* which means a greater state of self-clarity, happiness, and peace of mind.

So, what are you waiting for? Read on to find out what benefits you stand to reap from yoga and how to get started.

CHAPTER ONE

Types of Yoga

When walking into a yoga class, one of the things that you have to come with is a positive and open mindset. The truth is, just like any other exercise, there is no one-size-fits-all exercise in yoga. For you to reap the benefits that you are looking for, you have to be willing to try as many exercises as you can.

On certain days, you may be feeling like sweating it all out, and on others, you just want a yoga class in which you engage in poses that allows you to hold one position for longer so that you get a deeper stretch of your body, mind, and soul. With the many types of yoga, you can achieve what you are looking for without necessarily feeling as though you are being pushed to do it. Here are the different types of yoga for you to explore.

Hatha

This type of yoga is often perceived as a blanket term as far as yoga is concerned. It simply refers to the ability of one to link poses in between breaths. This type of yoga is often set to a much slower pace so that you can hold each pose for a prolonged duration of time.

As a beginner, Hatha classes are a great way to ease your mind and body into yoga, deepening your practice and expertise with time. This is mainly because, when you learn how to hold poses for longer, you allow yourself to sink deeper into each pose to achieve the required alignment.

Vinyasa

These classes are often fast-paced compared to the Hatha which is slower. With this type of yoga, the idea is for you to learn how to synchronize your movements with your breath. In other words, you learn how to work your way through a series of poses in a much more fluid manner.

With Vinyasa, you have a chance to engage in vigorous movements coupled with a flow from one posture to another. Therefore, if you are looking for a workout rather than just relaxation, Vinyasa is the one for you. It is dynamic and athletic, and that is a great deal for someone looking to sweat it out.

Ashtanga

This is a unique kind of yoga in which all the classes use a similar series of poses. This means that it is important for you to master the first series of poses before you proceed to the next one and the one after that. Therefore, if you are a perfectionist, this might just be the type of yoga that suits your personality better. However, before you get to Ashtanga, it is critical that you go through Vinyasa and Hatha first to master the art of synching your movements and breaths.

Yin yoga

This type of yoga requires that you master how to hold your poses for a couple of minutes at a time. In other words, you must know how to soften your muscles so that they can relax. The main aim is the deeper connective tissue and the fascia. This type of exercise is more meditative than others and explains why exercising this yoga helps relax both the mind and the muscles for a fuller, more satisfying well-being.

Bikram Yoga

This type of yoga is unique in the sense that it has a specific order of 26 posture and two breathing exercises. What is even more interesting about this kind of exercise is you practice it in a heated room. The main aim of the heat is to help the body relax, stretch deeper, release tension and stress, detox, and relieve chronic pain. Sometimes, the Vinyasa classes are also heated. However, when you think of hot yoga, what comes to mind is Bikram.

Kundalini

This is a type of yoga that is slightly different from all the others we have discussed. This is mainly because it incorporates a much more intense breath workout. It also has lots of meditations and chanting exercises. The main purpose of this is to help you elevate your consciousness while activating your body's energy centers or chakras.

CHAPTER TWO

Why you should practice yoga?

We live in a culture in which the mind and the nervous system is constantly stimulated. It is through yoga that you can slow down your mind so that you can restore your sanity and sense of balance. According to a study conducted in 2016, findings indicated that over 37 million people practiced Yoga around the world. Compared to 2012, this is a 50% increase.

Although the strength in numbers do not lie, the truth is that there is no clarity on the direct cause for this growth in yoga's popularity. But, we could think of this as a direct indicator of the benefits that this mindful practice offers to human life and health. It offers us benefits;

a) Physically
b) Spiritually
c) Mentally

Physical benefits of Yoga

One of the most obvious benefits of yoga is seen in the physical outlook. This is because it can increase one's strength, flexibility, balance, and mobility. This explains why so many athletes practice yoga as part of their effective cross-training program.

During yoga practice, one important thing to note is that the body goes through a wide range of motions that relieves pain and cramps in the body. Most of which is often a result of tensed up muscles or having poor postural habits. It is also through yoga that you become self-aware of your body. This self-awareness goes a long way in fixing any imbalances in your body and your athleticism is improved tremendously.

Yoga helps relieve stress and attain relaxation

This is one of the key benefits that yoga offers. Having gone through all the busyness of the week, there is a high chance that the body tends to accumulate stress. This causes the nervous system to have a constant overdrive that makes it hard to sleep, focus or even unwind. During yoga, the breathing exercises help you lower the heart rate so that the mind can shift to a more relaxed state. When you attain relaxation, you can get better sleep and focus more easily on your daily tasks.

On the other hand, if you are someone with a more spiritual background, the effects of yoga are often felt beyond the physical body. It is through yoga that you can begin to unravel your deeper sense of purpose and self-awareness. As you journey through your inner state of self, you begin to feel changes

take place based on what you need. You discover that you can now connect with yourself at a deeper level, the fruits of which are evident both inward and outwards.

One thing that you have to remember is that, no matter what you go through in life, what matters most is allowing yourself to feel what you feel. When you do so, you are in a better position to let go of what poisons the body so that you can have room for better things to strengthen you. The truth is, when you hold on tension, pain, fear, and trauma, you are in effect allowing mental distress to eat you up. This is not good for your health or perspective on life.

Yoga will help you release that tension from both your mind and body so that your overall health is improved. Ensure that you incorporate yoga to your daily routine to reap the benefits it has to offer to your mind and muscle recovery.

How can you quiet your mind with Yoga?

One thing to bear in mind is that Yoga is not only physically challenging, but also mentally. One of the hardest exercises that yoga has is learning how to quiet your mind in moments when everything needs to be still. Yes, we go through life with so many good things happening, but bad stuff also happens. Despite all the noise around us, how can we regain our inner peace and silence our minds?

While there are different yoga exercises and poses that can help you achieve this state of mind, almost all of them incorporate meditations and moments of stillness. Often, this part comes at the end of the exercise so you can wrap up your practice in a rather "*savasana*" manner.

Start by laying your yoga mat on the floor and then gently allow yourself to lie on your back in calm relaxation. At this point, your yoga instructor will start guiding you towards finding a quiet breathing pattern. Pay attention to the sound of your breath. This will help draw your focus and attention away from the busyness and noises of life so that you can find a mantra. In other words, you can find a phrase that you can keep repeating with your breath like "all is well" or "I am grateful" etc. When you find your mantra and start using it with your breathing, you will start to feel how soothing it is and hence helping you attain a state of relaxation and a peace of mind.

Just like meditation, it is critical that during a yoga class, you remember to allow your thoughts to come and go. Yes, we may have monkey minds with chaotic thoughts running around, but you can take control of what you think. Become your peaceful inner observer so that you can watch your thoughts as they come and go. When you learn how to quiet your mind, you will reap the health, physical and mental benefits that yoga has to offer.

What is the connection between yoga and spirituality?

This is a question that makes you feel like part of a yoga community. Even though so many yoga classes today teach lots of physical postures, the whole practice is not just an exercise. Some of the physical postures such as asana are one of the many limbs of yoga. The other limbs incorporate an entire system rooted in Hindu and Buddhism. It is through these practices that you learn how to govern your ethics, beliefs, behaviors, faith, and self-discipline. Through yoga exercises, you learn breathing, meditation and self-awareness.

Well, think about it; do you think that the yoga instructors just tell you how to stretch and bend and the class ends? No! The truth is, yoga exercises like asana were traditionally intended to help prepare the body for a much more divine spiritual growth, union, and discipline. This explains why yoga has a wide range of yogic texts and spiritual teachings derived from many faiths. However, don't get me wrong; yoga is not a religious meeting like some may think. It is surrounding in which people share experiences and discuss spirituality.

CHAPTER THREE

How do you as a beginner find the right class?

Step 1: Try before you start buying

Before you sign up for beginner classes, it is important that you know what is right for you. One of the most effective ways of getting started with yoga is identifying a beginner series at a local studio near you. Starting with entry level beginner classes is key to learning what to expect from a yoga class, understanding the basics, and then working through progressions with an instructor who is experienced in this.

What if my local studio does not have a beginner series? If this is the case, you don't have to worry. There are so many beginner sessions in many studios not far from where you live. The truth is, every studio has its own structure of classes which can be quite different from one another. Therefore, when you take multiple beginner classes, you get access to a variety of exercises which will keep you on your toes.

If you still cannot find a beginner class that you are comfortable with, you don't have to worry because each class has a series of progressions. This simply means that the yoga instructor will help guide you through different types of poses so that your body can begin to warm up. It is important that you speak with your teacher before classes start so that they can help guide you through the variations and start you on some beginner level poses. They will help you choose the right poses for you so that you can eventually learn to listen to your body while exercising patience.

Talk to your instructor or anyone on the yoga team at the studio to see whether you can have special introductory offers. Once you have gone through the classes for a month, there is a high chance that you will have a sense of direction on where to go next. You can make an informed choice of whether to commit your money and time into yoga or not. Trust me; sometimes just a single class is enough to help you understand the benefits you stand to reap from yoga practice.

Step 2: Practice from home

Sometimes, the idea of walking into a studio may sound intimidating at first when you are a beginner. If this is what you feel, you can start by practicing yoga at home. There are so many online yoga meditation classes you can sign up for and do them at the comfort of your home. Even YoutTube has an abundance of videos which can help you get started,

Another choice is **Yoga Glo,** who offers a 15-day free trial package for practices at all levels, irrespective of your experience. Well, this is just until you are comfortable to attend yoga classes in person. I encourage taking online classes just so that you know what to expect. In as much as online yoga lessons are comfortable, it is important that you establish a connection with a teacher so that you get to experience the progression in person.

Step 3: Try out different studios

Sometimes, it is hard to know which studio will offer the best experience that will help you connect with yourself at a deeper level. This is often a dilemma that most beginners have when they go into one studio, and they realize that it is not meeting their needs and expectations.

Therefore, before you can commit to a yoga studio for beginner classes, it is important that you sign up for introductory classes just to get a feel of what they have to offer. You can even stop by and talk to the yoga team. In the same way, gyms run yoga studios and have a wide range of fitness goals and programs. Getting a feel of what options each studio has to offer helps you make an informed choice on one that you feel better connected to. Sample their styles, instructors, and service.

Some of what you should look out for when sampling include the following;

Location and cost

This might seem like a no-brainer but is one of the most critical factors to consider when looking for a yoga class to attend. The truth is, regardless of whether you sign up for the best in town, location is a big deal. If the location and the cost are prohibitive, it can be very hard to establish a routine that is practical for you.

Community

This is one of the factors that is most overlooked by many beginners. However, the community of the yoga studio you want has to be good enough to contribute towards your experience and growth. The truth is, a yoga class alone is not fun at all. You need to practice with others to get that wonderful experience.

Part of the whole benefit is for you to learn how to engage with others in life. If you have no community, you start feeling lonely and empty inside. When trying to figure out what yoga community you would like to join, these questions will help you make an informed choice;

- What kind of social life are you interested in? Do you intend to interact with people from your yoga class or would you just want to take the class and leave? Would you want a studio with a coffee shop so that you grab a coffee with a friend after to have a more social experience?

- Do you intend to learn more about meditation, natural health, and nutrition from your yoga lessons? Are you interested in traditional or more modernized fitness classes?
- Are you interested in making spirituality part of your exercise? This is because, some studios just teach asana; which is a physical posture for exercise. Others are interested in teaching reflections, meditations, and chanting.

What classes are offered?

Well, the truth is, location and community are the most important factors to consider when choosing a studio for your beginner yoga lessons. However, you are not going to be a beginner forever. If you intend to keep yoga as part of your lifestyle, you should think about the future. You must think long-term!

This is why you have to consider what classes the yoga studio you choose has to offer. This means that, as your practice grows, you will have access to more challenging classes or have classes that specifically target areas that you feel limited. Whatever it is, always look at the bigger picture!

Step 4: Finding the right yoga instructor

One of the questions that many beginners ask is "how do I find the right yoga teacher?" Well, the truth is, finding the right teacher depends on what you are looking for. You should pay attention to finding a teacher that connects with you. Someone with whom you feel you resonate with from the moment you set foot in a studio. Whenever they are coaching, you feel like they are talking to you.

When you go for your very first introductory class, it should be about finding a teacher that you can connect with, irrespective of the styles and poses taught. If you are going to reap the benefits of yoga from a class, then you will have to have someone that is straight up with you. You need that one person that will pay attention to your needs and give you feedback after practice.

Additionally, as I said earlier, you are not going to be a beginner forever! Therefore, you need a teacher that will help you grow, and the best way to grow is through the challenge. Your practice should meet you where you are and not at the destination. When you are trying to find the right instructor, ask yourself, "what do I feel around them?", "Do I like how I feel whenever I am around them in class and outside class?" If the teacher is what you would like to resemble after a long time of practice, then that is who you are looking for.

But while you're at it, you have to bear in mind that yoga is an inner journey that is unique to you. It is not just a physical practice like any other. Therefore, if you are going to get in touch with your inner self, you need an instructor you are free with. Someone that you feel safe and comfortable around. Ensure that the teacher you settle for is one that encourages you to be better. Someone that pushes you to go on and push out of your comfort zone. In other words, the right teacher is that one person that gives you the need to keep on with practice to self-study.

Step 5: Always start with a beginner class even if you are not a beginner

You may have dabbled in some yoga practice at home through videos and online classes, which you have learned all the basic poses. The question is "do you still sign up for beginner classes?" Well, the shortest answer is; YES!

The truth is, having some experience with yoga exercises does not mean that you have mastered all you need to for you to attend a more advanced class. Being in a yoga class environment is key in helping you push through your limits. You also need to connect with your instructor. Just skipping the beginner classes for an intermediate class can be too much for you to handle and you might end up giving up before you even get started.

Indeed, there is a blurry line between what is a beginner class and an intermediate yoga class. However, the best person to tell you what level you are is not your instructor, but you. It comes down to what you feel. Is the class you are in manageable? Is it challenging? Do you feel more lost in class compared to your colleagues?

One thing that you have to remember is that advancing to the next stage does not necessarily mean that you cannot come back to the beginner class. Even though I am advanced, I still go to beginner classes. This is where you get the time to let your mind settle, move with extreme intentions while ensuring that your mindset is meditative.

For the best classroom experience, it is important that you come early so that you have time to interact with your instructor. This makes it quite easy for them to teach you better especially when they know you are a beginner. Additionally, if you have any underlying health conditions, it is best that you let your instructor know before you get started. This way, they can make modifications to the poses to suit your condition. You do not want to exercise postures that will make your health condition worse!

Step 6: Ease into your yoga habits

Now that you know the right teacher and the best studio for you, the next thing is for you to start feeling comfortable. You want a yoga class that is supportive and inclusive. You want a chance to explore your practices without necessarily feeling like people are judging your technical abilities, clothes, and body. The truth is, your yoga classes will be worth your time and money if you reap the benefits and realize your goals. If not, it is time you look for another studio and instructor.

Your action plan should be;

- Make a list of all studios within places that are convenient for you. Ensure that they are not just close enough, but also affordable to increase your chances of going.
- Visit a couple of these studios and get their schedule and then start trying them out to get the vibe.
- Attempt a couple of beginner classes with different yoga instructors. At this point, it is not important that you commit to one instructor or style. Throughout practice, try out different styles, new classes, and instructors.
- Finally, show up in class early so that you can have a little chat with your instructor, especially if you have health concerns to share. When you follow this basic plan, you will start to feel more comfortable and have a fuller experience each time.

CHAPTER FOUR

Your Yoga Essentials

When starting yoga classes, you are not sure what to buy and what not to buy. This is because, when you walk into a fitness store, you will find so many yoga items, equipment, and clothing that might confuse you. These items are often very expensive and may discourage you even before you set foot in a yoga studio for your first class.

The good news is that, just like any other business, the yoga complex keeps growing with all these sophisticated items. All you need is very little.

Here are your essentials;

Clothing

For most yoga studios, it is a requirement that you are in the right attire in class. However, you do not need a score for your clothing. You do not need to have the designer gear to feel like part of the yoga community. It is important that you just start with something that you feel comfortable in. Clothing that is breathable and other mid-level basics to start you off.

You need;

Pants/shorts

When starting as a beginner, having a few pairs of solid color pants is a plus. You can then mix and match them up with a wide variety of tops. Ensure that you get something that is of good quality so that they can last even longer.

If you cannot get yoga pants, go for jogger-style pants or harem pants instead. Ensure that the ankles are elastic enough. These kind of pants are usually breathable and have elastic ankles to stay in place throughout practice.

For men, yoga shorts are quite a popular option. They are also worn by women nowadays especially when in a hot yoga class. Just ensure that you are in form-fitting spandex shorts or shorts that are loose with tights underneath for those poses that are quite uncomfortable.

Tops

It is critical that you have tops that are fairly fitting to hold your bust in place when you bend forward. If you are prone to sweating or plan to attend a hot yoga class, wicking materials are superior to others. Additionally, since yoga rooms are often kept cool, you may find it useful to carry along a light sweater so that you wear it until your class begins.

Hair ties

If you have long hair, it is important that you have a good hair tie to secure them in place during practice. Some poses require you to bend forward, sideways and all over and having your hair falling on your eyes and face can make the whole experience quite distracting.

Yoga socks

This is not a requirement for you to be in class, but it is something that makes your feet feel comfortable rather than exercising on barefoot. However, some people are not comfortable with strangers looking at their feet. If you are this kind of person, then a pair of socks with a good grip can come in handy. The grip at the bottom of the socks ensures that you maintain good traction. Never exercise in standard socks because they are slippery and you might end up falling and getting injured.

Yoga Mat

This is one of the most important items when in a yoga class. It is often referred to as a sticky mat. It is that thing that will define your personal space in class. It also plays a significant role in creating traction on both your feet and hands so that you do not slip and fall when you are a little sweaty. It's also important in providing cushioning on a hard floor, hence making practice comfortable.

Most yoga studios provide their mats for rent at a small fee. This is usually fine if it is your very first class/introductory classes before you figure out what mats are good. However, it is advisable that you have a mat of your own considering others are used by many people and you cannot be certain of their state of hygiene.

Indeed, premium yoga mats can be costly, but you can get a starter mat for around $20 at Target or on Amazon. The disadvantage of getting a cheap mat is that you have to replace it within a short time because of quick wear and tear. If you have made up your mind to do yoga long-term, a yoga mat is something worth spending your cash on.

When purchasing a yoga mat, there are several factors that you have to consider. Some of these factors include the length, material, and thickness of the mat. It is also critical that you get a material that is durable, comfortable and has traction on both your feet and hands. Additionally, you want something easy to clean. You can check out product reviews before buying to learn the experiences that others have had using a similar kind. This will help you make an informed choice.

Optional Equipment

There are a wide range of items that are not at the top of your list of priorities, but are good to have if you have the budget for them. Some of these items include;

Yoga props

Props are known to play a role in helping maintain a healthy alignment when on a wide range of poses. This includes when you bend, open up or twist. They are important in helping you make the most of every exercise without necessarily injuring yourself. It is important that you familiarize yourself with them before you purchase.

Blocks

Just like blankets, yoga blocks are also meant to offer you extra comfort and alignment. This is especially the case when on a standing pose that requires your hands on the floor. Having blocks under your hands makes the floor slightly raised, e.g., When you are doing a half-moon pose. It also offers your hamstring flexibility and core strength that helps you hold your position with proper form. Additionally, when you place a block under your arms, you can easily keep your torso strong and chest open, hence maintaining proper alignment. Most Yoga blocks are made of cork, wood or foam.

They are also adaptable, especially when made to stand at different heights. If you are doing yoga at home, it is advisable that you get a set of blocks. However, if you are attending yoga studio classes, then these will be provided for you.

Mat bags/slings

If you have a yoga mat, then you are going to be carrying it with you to the studio and back regularly. Having a mat bag or a sling can come in handy in keeping your mat in good condition and making transport easy.

If you choose to go for a sling, it is important to note that they often come with Velcro straps which allows you to bind your rolled mat with a connecting strap to throw it on your shoulder. They also have extra storage pockets for anything else you might want to carry with you.

On the other hand, bags come in two styles; one that uses Velcro straps to keep the rolled mat in position on a gym bag. The other is a zipper bag that is designed specifically to hold the rolled mat on its own. Both have extra storage for anything you might want to bring with you like cell phones, wallets, and changing clothes.

Blankets

Many studios have stacks of blankets for students when they need to use one. You can use them to support you as you lift your hips while on a sitting position or when lying on the floor. The truth is, they play a key role as far as different yoga exercises are concerned. You can also use them to cover yourself up during final relaxation if the room is quite chilly. For the sake of hygiene, it is better if you can get a blanket of your own if you find it necessary to have one. You can grab one at home if you have extra that you can spare for yoga practice.

Bolsters

This is something that you can use in place of a blanket to make your alignments comfortable. You can use them under your knees or back so that you get support when reclining and when stretching. If you are recovering from an injury or are pregnant, bolsters are your closest friends.

Bolsters come in two shapes; flat and round. The flat ones often are ergonomic while the round ones are critical when you need extra support when stretching deeper. It is all about your taste and preference. If you do not have any preference, you can use both depending on what you would like to achieve.

Straps

They are also referred to as belts. They are specifically useful for poses that need you to hold your feet, but you cannot reach them. The straps serve as extensions to your arms. For instance, when doing the pascimottasana pose, you can simply wrap the strap at the bottom of your feet and then hold onto them so that the back is flat and not bent forward.

You can also use them when you need to bind your arms around your back in cases where your shoulders are not flexible enough for the bind. Sometimes, you do not need to buy one. At home, you may have something like a belt or a towel that you can bring with you to the studio for use during a yoga class.

CHAPTER FIVE

How do you prepare for your first Yoga class?

Ensure that you have the right clothing

When attending a yoga class, it is important that you are in the right gear. It is advisable that you wear layers on top of your gear if it's cold outside. When it gets too hot, you can shed them off one by one. Also, consider the various poses that you engage in during practice so that you do not feel too tight when doing downward dog; or too loose when riding up.

Ensure that what you are wearing is comfortable so that you can focus on what your instructor is telling you rather than worrying whether your knickers are flashing out or your boobs are falling out of your bras.

Men, unlike women, have a limited choice of yoga clothing. The good thing is that you do not have to worry too much about what top to wear if you are comfortable without one. On the other hand, choosing the right pants can be tricky, and if you are not careful, they may hinder you from exercising comfortably.

Take off your socks

As mentioned earlier, yoga is practiced with bare feet. However, at the beginning of the class, you might want to keep them on if the weather is cold. Your instructor will advise you when to take them off. You can also buy socks with a grip if you do not want to workout barefoot.

Try as much as you can to stick to your yoga mat and not topple over to another person's mat. Many people regard their mat as their personal space and not just a piece of rubber, and the last thing you want is invading someone's personal space.

Grab something light to eat before class

It is not a good idea to start exercising on an empty stomach. On the other hand, it is also not advisable to exercise when your stomach is full. Ensure that you at least have something light before practice like a banana or yogurt because some exercises might be challenging and you need all the strength and flexibility you can get.

Familiarize with some yoga terms

Some instructors like using yoga pose in Sanskrit. However, you do not have to worry because most of them use English and you can ask them to translate when you do not understand. To avoid any confusion, it is important that you at least learn common yogic texts and keep up as time goes by.

Learn to keep to your space

Remember when I mentioned that some people regard their yoga mats as personal species? Well, this is very true and a sense of ownership exhibited by many! Before heading for your first class, ensure that you practice at home just to familiarize yourself with using your mat as your personal space and not toppling over to another's area.

One thing that you should note is that most yoga studios have several people attending one class. This means that, if the room is not that large, you might end up each being on a 5 cm apart. This might feel strange at first, but with time, you will get used to it. Yoga can be quite difficult to practice when space is limited, especially when someone is hovering over your face. Just learn to stick to your area.

Your edge

When you are a beginner, it may be hard to differentiate between discomfort and pain. Well, pain can be defined as a sudden sharp sensation, and you might not feel it during exercise. However, you might feel a little discomfort; a sensation that is rather nagging and often changes when you breathe into it. Just remember that you are your best instructor. In other words, you know exactly where you feel the discomfort better than anyone around you. Therefore, you know when it is a cause for alarm or when it is just a small pinch. Learn to listen to your body so that you do not push yourself over the edge.

Learn how to chant

You will realize that some classes will entail chanting with people saying "Om- Om." Anyways, some of these chants may be shorter while others are longer with calls and responses, which you might find strange at first. If you do not wish to join in, that is fine.

However, one thing that is important to note is that chanting can be fun and wonderful at the same time. It is a way in which you join in with the rest of the crew in uniting your energy as a group. Some will even include you folding your arms at your heart with heads bowed down and mouths uttering "Namaste" which simply means that the light within me bows to the light within you.

Remember to breathe

The whole idea of yoga is to help you connect with your breath and inner self. This explains why your instructor will guide you through a series of breathing exercises such as pranayama. Your instructor will be giving instructions on how to do it, however, the secret is for you to keep breathing the whole time.

Indeed, this can be confusing at first. You might find yourself breathing in when you are supposed to be breathing out and the other way around. However, you do not have to worry much. Keep practicing, and soon everything will begin to fall in place effortlessly.

Take control of your emotions

One of the things that we learn during yoga practice is to become aware of ourselves. In other words, you have to get in touch with your inner self for you to feel your body. This has an impact on helping our subconscious minds get a place of safety so that the whole body can start to relax. When we start to let go of the physical tension, we can experience our emotions being released with them.

The truth is, at some point, you might experience a strong emotion during yoga. It may be feelings of frustrations, joy, sadness, tears and being vulnerable. Do not fear to allow your emotions to get released as this is something very normal (and a sign that you're growing from within). Try as much as you can not to pass judgments. Allow them to be what they are - emotions!

It's also important that you remain respectful of those around you who may be undertaking a similar experience. The communities created within yoga groups are often built on emotions and deep connections can be bonded. If the practice houses a café or coffee house, why not join them for a drink after to draw on each other's experiences.

Leave your ego outside

Some people think that yoga is athletics where you are competing against each other. Unlike other sports, yoga is not competitive, hence the reason why you should leave your self-criticism and ego outside.

Additionally, when you need the support of props, blankets, and belts among other things, use them. Don't fear that people will think of you as a beginner at the expense of your comfort during practice. Think of it as a way of getting more space while on a pose as well as allowing you to get better alignment.

On the other hand, if you need to rest at some point during class, rest! One of the essential rules of yoga is Ahimsa which simply translates to "no harm." Therefore, when you start with that in mind, this means that you are also careful not to cause harm on yourselves or others whether physically, emotionally or mentally. Just exercise a lot of kindness, and that will transform your social interactions and mindset positively.

Take part in Savasana

This is the relaxation session of a yoga class. It can also be one of the most challenging parts of yoga, especially for a beginner which is why so many people skip it altogether. It is important that you take part in. You may be thinking "who has time to lie around?"

Well, it is important that you start how you think and your general perspective of life. This is mainly because Savasana allows you to absorb the benefits of each posture. Think of it as your rest button. It's where you go to when you need to calm your mind and nervous system. It is where you bring your breathing and heart rate to be normal. It is where you just allow yourself to be you without worrying about what others might think of us.

Always come with your beginner mind

This is referred to as *Shoshin*. This is a term derived from Zen Buddhism that simply means approaching everything with an open mind and eagerness. Rather than coming to a yoga class with preconceptions, it is important that we come with a beginner's mind. The truth is, you cannot be that bad at it even though there will always be someone more flexible or stronger than us.

You will not master everything all at once. Most of the poses will need your patience and commitment. It is also critical that you demonstrate respect for your body's limits so that you know when you are pushing too far and when you are not pushing enough. Learn how to connect with your emotions and breath so you can be present in every moment. Rather than getting angry and frustrated when you cannot balance a tree pose for a couple of minutes, just let loose and enjoy the experience. Remember, practice makes perfect!

CHAPTER SIX

Beginner poses to expect

Below are a number of poses which you can expect to learn as a beginner, which you'll also be taught during classes. You should read through the descriptions below, then search videos and photos on the Internet for a visual reference. Google and YouTube will be great resources on your yoga journey.

Mountain Pose

This is also referred to as Tadasana. The term "Tada" simply means mountain, hence the name mountain pose. It teaches you how to stand with a majestic steadiness, just like a mountain does. While using this pose, you are required to use a major group of muscles so that you can boost your concentration and focus. It is considered a starting position for all other asana poses.

Start by standing with your heels slightly apart. Then hang your arms on your sides adjacent to your torso. Begin to lift and spread the toes gently so that the balls of your feet are steady and elevated. Then lay them on the floor mat softly so that your body weight is balanced on your feet.

Now, lift your ankles and firm your thigh muscles in such a way that they start rotating inwards. As you begin to inhale, elongate your torso. Then exhale while releasing your shoulder blades away from your head. While doing this, ensure that your collarbone is broadened and the neck elongated.

While on this pose, one of the things that you have to bear in mind is that the ears, ankles, hips, and shoulders have to be aligned together. The best way to check your alignment is when standing against a wall at first. You could also raise your hands and stretch them out while allowing your breath to come easy.

Downward Facing Dog

This is also referred to as the Adho Mukha Svanasana. This is one of the most popular yoga poses, and it plays a critical role in helping stretch and strengthen the whole body. An old yoga saying is, 'a downward dog each day, will help keep the doctor away!'

Start by laying your yoga mat straight on the floor. Now, begin coming on to all fours with your wrists straight under your shoulders so that the hips are positioned directly under the hips. Slowly tuck yourself under your toes. Begin to lift your hips from the mat and draw them back to your heels.

While keeping your knees slightly bent so that your hamstrings are loosened, try and straighten out your legs while maintaining your hips behind. Start walking your hands forward to get more extension if need be.

Using your palms, press firmly against the floor so that your inner elbows rotate slightly and move towards each other. Keep engaging your legs so that your torso is not moving back to your thighs, hence allowing you to hollow your abdominals. Without changing position, hold your breath for a couple of minutes and then slowly drop to your hands and knees for a rest.

Crescent Lunge

This is also referred to as the Utthita Ashwa Sanchalanasa. With this pose, the first thing that you do is to take a giant step forward using your left foot so that you are in a staggered stance. Ensure that your feet are almost the length of the mat apart. Bend the front knee while maintaining the back leg straight. Lift your heel off the floor and then try bending your front leg forward. Ensure that your thigh is parallel to the floor.

Once you are in position, square your hips to the front and then extend your arms towards the ceiling on both sides, stretch upwards while ensuring that your feet press into the mat and the stretch is felt on your hips. Hold that position for a couple of minutes and then repeat the same on the other side.

On the other hand, if you want to move into the low lunge; or what is otherwise referred to as Anjaneyasana pose, all you have to do is drop your back knee and shin onto the mat while ensuring that you keep the leg extended. When on this pose, one of the critical things to consider is keeping the spine long than it is so that your back leg is straightened well. Also, you are at liberty to bend the back leg if you need support when lifting your torso so that the back is extended.

You have to note that, different instructors often have different interpretations of the various lunge poses. The other will refer to it as crescent lunge while others call it high lunge, but they are all the same thing with hands placed on the mat on both sides of the front leg.

Warrior II

This is also referred to as Virabhadrasana II. The first thing you do is take a big step forward using your left foot so that you are in a staggered position with your feet apart. Then start extending your arms outwards to the side so that they are parallel to the floor. Bend the knee so that it is at a right angle with the thigh parallel to the floor. Ensure that the right leg is maintained straight.

Start pointing the left toes to the front while turning the right foot out to the right orientation until it is perpendicular to the left leg. Ensure that the left heel is aligned with the right foot's arch. At the same time, slightly twist your torso towards the right direction in such a way that the left hip is facing towards the front of the room and the right hip facing backward. The left arm and head should point forward while the right arm points backward. In that position, hold your breath for a couple of minutes.

Tip: ensure that the left knee does not move past the ankle because this would cause a slight reduction in the depth of the lunge.

Triangle

This is also referred to as Trikonasana. This is one of the most popular yoga poses that is characterized by standing so that the sides of the waist are stretched and the longs are opened. It also strengthens the legs and tones the whole body.

To do it, start by standing straight on your feet with the legs a length apart. Now, open your arms to the sides so that they are at the height of your shoulders. Turn the right foot at a right angle and the left toes in like 45°. While hinging to sides and over the right leg, engage the quadriceps and the abdominals. Ensure that your right hand is placed on the ankle, knee or shin so that the left arm is lifted straight to the ceiling.

Direct your gaze towards the top hand and then in that position, hold your breath for a couple of minutes. Lift yourself to a standing position and repeat the whole process on the other side. To be successful in this pose, imagine yourself stuck in between two walls when in a triangle.

Chair Pose

This is also referred to as the Kursiasana. This is an intensely powerful pose that plays a significant role in helping strengthen both your leg and arm muscles. It is a pose that goes a long way in building your willpower leaving your body and mind feeling energized.

Start by standing with your feet a little bit apart from each other. Then stretch your arms without bending the elbows. Now, inhale while bending your knees and pushing your pelvis down as though you are sitting on a chair. Ensure that you keep the rams parallel to the floor and your back as straight as can be. Begin to take in deep breaths while gradually bending and keeping the knees above and behind your toes.

Boat Pose

This is also referred to as the Naukasana pose. It plays a central role in tightening the abdominal muscles. It is also important in strengthening the upper back and the shoulders, and hence can increase your sense of stability.

To do this, start by lying on your mat with your back in contact with the floor. Put your feet together and your hands straight on the side. Take deep breathes and every time you exhale, do so gently such that your chest and feet are lifted off the floor. Ensure that while doing this, your hands are stretched towards your feet. Additionally, your eyes, toes, and fingers should be aligned together.

Hold that position for as long as you can until there is some tension in the navel area, and the abdomen begins to contract. As you exhale, bring your whole body back to the floor while exhaling and allowing yourself to relax.

Cobra Pose

This is also referred to as the Bhujangasana pose. This pose plays a very significant role in helping strengthen the lower back muscles while ensuring that the spine, chest and the triceps are well cushioned for proper inhalation. It also boosts the flexibility of the spine.

Start by lying on your stomach with both feet together and the toes flat on the mat. Then move your hands downwards so that they are positioned slightly below the shoulders on the mat. Now, lift your waist and then raise your head while breathing in slowly and gently.

Then pull your torso back while supporting them with your hands. Ensure that you maintain your elbows straight so that both palms have equal pressure pushing on them. Slowly tilt your head backward and ensure that your shoulders are far from your ears. Slowly exhale and allow your body to come back to the floor.

Seated forward fold

This is referred to as the *Paschimottanasana*. It is an asana pose that plays a critical role in boosting the hamstring's flexibility and that of the hip region. It is also important in lengthening the spine. Start by sitting up so that your back is straight and so that the toes are pointing outwards. Then start inhaling while raising your hands over your head and then stretch.

Now, as you exhale, move your hands downwards and bend forward so that you can touch your legs. Try to touch your toes, but don't push to a point where you'll cause injury to yourself. Alternatively, you can choose to place your hands right where they can reach. Then inhale in a while elongating your spine. As you exhale, ensure that your navel is as close to your knees as possible.

Child's pose

Similar to a child's feelings of innocence and helplessness, this posture helps you surrender and let go of anything that might be holding you back. It is one of the poses that plays a significant role in helping restore your vitality emotionally, mentally and physically. You can add this pose in the middle of other challenging asana poses to add some relaxation and focus.

Try this while closing your eyes so that you pay attention to your breathing. Try to bend your knees and sit on your heels. Ensure that you keep those knees on the heels as you lower your head towards the mat and then bring your hands towards the sides. Then gradually press your thighs against your chest and inhale gently.

Sukhasna

This is one of the most comfortable poses suitable for meditation and pranayama. It is through this posture that one can achieve a centering effect. The difference between this and the other asana poses is the fact that other poses are aimed at making the body eventually feel comfortable so that they can sit in a meditation position.

However, this pose helps the body stretch beyond its physical dimension because it helps you get in touch with your spiritual person. The first thing that you have to do is lay on your mat straight on the floor and sit comfortably with your legs crossed. Ensure that the left leg is tucked inside the right thigh such that the right leg is tucked under the left thigh. Ensure that the spine is maintained in a straight position. Now, let your hands rest on your knees and allow your body to relax as you inhale gently.

Plank Pose

This is also referred to as the Kumbkhakasana. Start by laying on all fours on your yoga mat so that your knees are under your hips. Ensure that your hands are flat on the mat, just parallel to your shoulders. Now, try to lift your knees above the ground while extending your legs so that they are out and behind you. At this point, you should be on your toes and hands, so that the whole body is in one line.

Now, keep the palms flat on the ground and the hands shoulder-width apart. Ensure that your shoulders are stacked above the wrists and the cores well engaged. Your spine and neck should be in a neutral position so that you look down on your mat. Maintain this position for about three minutes while holding your breath as well. Then let your whole body come to rest on your yoga mat.

Low Plank

This is also referred to as the Chaturanga Dandasana. To do this pose, start with the plank pose that we have discussed above while ensuring that your palms are flat on the mat. Your hands should be shoulder width apart and the shoulders stacked right above the wrists. Additionally, ensure that the legs are extended and your cores are well engaged.

Now, lower your body down to a low plank pose by bending your elbows so that they are tucked in somewhere close to the sides at a right angle. Hold your breath for a minute and exhale while bringing yourself to a resting position.

One thing that you have to note is that this pose is often preceded by an Upward-facing dog. It is important that you keep your shoulders above your elbow height. The truth is, if you cannot get it right the first time, there is no shame if you try to move away from your knees to maintain a stable posture.

Upward-facing dog

This is also referred to as the Urdhva Mukha Svanasana. It is easier to follow this pose soon after the low plank pose that we have discussed above. Start by dropping down on your hips and then twist your toes so that the top of your feet are in contact with the floor. Now, start tightening your core while strengthening your arms so that your chest is pushed up.

Begin to pull your shoulders back while squeezing the blades. Then tilt your head toward the ceiling so that your chest is opened up as much as possible. While exercising this pose, you should feel free to drop on your knees so that the tension exerted on your back is significantly reduced. You could also skip the upward-facing dog, or high plank poses altogether.

Half Pigeon Pose

This is also referred to as Ardha Kapotasana. Once you are through with the downward-facing dog, you can follow up with half pigeon pose. Start by extending your left leg high while bringing your body underneath it. Place the leg right in front of you so that your shin is parallel to the ground.

Now, start extending the right leg backward so that it is behind you. Then rest the top of your foot on the ground. Ensure that at this point, you maintain the left foot flexed. Additionally, try as much as you can to keep your right hip close to the floor as much as you can. This is because, if you lift it off the ground, you might lose your balance. Otherwise, if it lifts off the mat for some reason, bring your left foot slightly close to your body to achieve stability and balance.

Stay in this position for about five breaths and then fold over so that your head rests on the mat for another five breaths or so. Repeat the whole exercise with the other leg. In case you experience pain on your knees while in this pose, try to do reclined figure four. All you have to do is lie on your back and then bring your left foot over the right thigh so that the left foot is flexed.

Tree Pose

It is also referred to as the Vrksasana pose. This precedes the mountain pose so that your knees are brought together and the heels are apart from each other a little bit. Start by bringing you right foot towards your inner left thigh. Then squeeze your foot and the inner left thigh together as much as you can. Your left knee should be slightly twisted out so that the right thigh faces down at a 45° angle.

Once you have established some sort of stability, begin to bring your hands high to a prayer position right at the front of your chest. You could also bring them high such that they are overhead if this position works well for you. Pick a point right in front of you and gaze at it so that you can achieve some balance. Hold your breath for a couple of minutes before slowly switching to the other side.

Tip: If you find it difficult to achieve balance, try bringing your right foot over your left shin rather than the thigh.

Dancers Pose

This is also referred to as the Natarajasana.

Start by standing tall with both feet kept together. Slightly bend the left knee so that your left foot is positioned towards your glutes. Now, begin to grab onto your left foot's inner arch using your left hand and then slowly lift your left foot to the front and towards the ceiling. Simultaneously, try to reach out to your right arm at the front and upwards.

Using your right foot, actively press down into the yoga mat as you begin to open your chest and pull your leg up. Ensure that you keep the chest lifted and open. In that position, hold your breath for a couple of minutes before you can switch to the other side to repeat the whole exercise.

One of the things that you have to bear in mind is for you to focus on keeping your hips at a level rather than bringing your foot high. This will go a long way in keeping your lower back in a comfortable position while avoiding overstretching yourself too much.

CHAPTER SEVEN

Do's and Do Not's of Yoga

Do's

Hydrate as much as you can

One of the things that you have to remember at all times is that water is life! Therefore, if you have a yoga class planned, it is important that you keep hydrating throughout the day.

It is advisable that you do not drink water throughout the yoga lesson unless you are practicing hot yoga. This is because, during hot yoga, you will be losing lots of water from the body and you need to drink up to stay hydrated and focused.

Consult with your medical Doctor

Before you engage in any intense physical activity such as yoga, ensure that you have discussed it with your doctor. This is especially important if you have had or have an injury or prevailing health conditions.

Yes, many people think of yoga as a cure that cannot harm you. Despite this, it is important that your doctor gives you the go-ahead to avoid any accidents happening. Otherwise, there are many minds, body, and soul benefits of yoga and you should take advantage of them while you still can.

Fill in your yoga instructor if you have injuries or health conditions

One of the most important things when it comes to any workouts is safety. It is critical that you inform your yoga instructor of any injuries you might have had or any health conditions. Additionally, if you are pregnant, it is important that you let your teacher know. Some instructors will ask you while signing up for the class while others will not. Therefore, if they don't ask, approach them and let them know.

One of the key roles of a teacher is to ensure that the students are comfortable during sessions. This includes modifying some of the exercises to suit their condition. If they do not know your current condition or previous medical history, they might just treat you like the rest of the class, and that means the exercises might be vigorous and unintentionally impact your condition.

Most of the teachers also have assistants so you can let them know of your condition if you are not as comfortable with your instructor. They are often the ones giving hands-on modifications, and it is important they are aware so that they can help you.

Know your edge

Your body is yours, and only you know what it wants. One of the things that you should know is when your body has had enough, and that is where you stop. While practicing yoga, it is critical that you push yourself so that you can keep making progress. However, you should know when to press the stop or pause button if it hurts or puts you at risk of injury.

The truth is, it often takes time before one can get their perfect balance. This is because it takes time for anyone to learn how to get back and reconnect with the body. Bear in mind, experiencing some mild discomfort is okay. However, when you start to feel some sharp pain in the joints, it could be a sign that you are hurting yourself and pushing your body to extremes. At this point, what you need to do is to gently back off so that you do not cause more harm than good. Your body needs to rest before it can resume. Give it that! A little TLC will not hurt.

Be gentle when having your menses (women)

Yoga during menstruation can be a great way of relieving pain. However, it is also essential that you take things a little easy on yourself. You could do this by either attending hatha or some therapeutic form of yoga rather than engaging in vigorous exercises and poses.

Traditionally, it was thought that skipping inversions during menstruation would be helpful. Rather than putting a pause altogether, you could make a few adjustments to your yoga poses to help you make the most of your time. You could modify and do leg-up-the wall pose. You should pay close attention to the needs of your body and do what feels right at that moment.

Be in a comfortable gear

If there is something distracting you during workouts then you should reconsider your apparel. Ensure that what you wear is comfortable, breathable and free to stretch. Something that will technically not restrain your movements nor get in the way of exercising.

If you plan on attending slowly paced classes such as Yin and Hatha, it is advisable that you pack something loose and light. Ensure that your clothing, whether it be; leggings, tops, shorts, or even bras are fitting and comfortable for such classes as Ashtanga or Vinyasa.

Trust me, yoga is not about looking all pretty. Rather, it is about ensuring that you are not distracted by anything so that all your focus is on your instructor and doing what you are instructed to do. You don't want to injure yourself because you wore something that got in the way during exercise.

It is advisable that you wear formfitting gear so that it is easier for your instructor to tell when you are aligned and when you are not. Additionally, if you predict that it might get chilly during Savasana class, try to carry a hoodie or a sweater with you to keep you warm.

Take a bath before class

One thing that you have to bear in mind is that cleanliness inside and out is key when it comes to yoga. Taking a shower before class will make you feel fresh. It is also this simple gesture that will demonstrate that you have respect for your instructor and students. Body odors can be very distracting!

Leave your shoes at the door

Another way of practicing the principle of saucha in yoga is by taking off your shoes before you step into the yoga room. This is because, much of the workouts you will engage in will be closer to the floor, and the last thing you want is breathing close to a dusty, muddy floor. Therefore, leaving your shoes by the door ensures that your space is dirt and germ-free.

You may be thinking "what if it is cold?" Well, if you feel the room is chilly, you can keep your socks on as you come in and take them off later once the class starts. You could also choose to have non-slip yoga socks that you can wear throughout the class.

When you need a break, take it

So many people often think that the downward dog is not a resting pose and if you feel this way, you can choose to do a child's pose whenever you feel that you need a rest during practice. The bottom line is for you to pay attention to what your body wants and give it just that!

Put away your props after practice

If you take your yoga lessons at the studio and use several shared equipment or items, it is important that you put them back after practice. It does not only ensure that they are kept in good condition, but also shows respect to the staff and your fellow students who are going to be using them after you are done.

Don'ts

Come to class late

Your yoga instructors ensure that they plan their classes early enough. This means that when you come in late, you miss parts of it and lose the benefits of a comfortable and thought out session. You also don't get to warm up like the rest of the class to bring your body up to speed (leading to a greater risk of injury).

It is important that you come in 15 minutes before the class begins. This is the time that you will use to unwind and change into your yoga clothes without necessarily having to rush. You can also roll out your mat and anything else you might need during class. You will also have a chance to take a few minutes of quiet time on your mat to self-reflect before class.

Of course, some things are inevitable and if something happens and you cannot avoid being late, ensure that you let your instructor know. When you finally join, do it quietly to avoid causing the rest of the class any distractions.

Skip Savasana

This is one of the sessions that most students skip because they think it is has the hardest poses. This is mainly because we find it hard to lie down and do nothing! It is a great way for you to relieve stress. It offers the body an opportunity to achieve total relaxation before we can get back to the busyness of our lives.

Additionally, if you intend on establishing a schedule for meditation practice, this is the best place to start. Indeed, it may be challenging at first, but if you stick with it, you will have yourself to thank later.

Engage your neighbor in a conversation

One of the most important things when it comes to yoga is space. It is critical that you respect your space and that of others during practice. The other thing is that you should not be engaging your neighbor in conversation during class. If it is time for yoga, focus on what your instructor says and take up a conversation with your neighbor after class.

By talking to them during class, you are not just distracting them and others, but also disrespecting your instructor. If what you would like to say to them cannot wait until after class, you can ask your instructor by raising your hand or giving them a gesture. The last thing you want is attracting the whole class' attention.

Judge others and yourself

Yoga is an exercise that is free of any judgments. The truth is, it does not matter what you or others wear during practice or how you are doing the poses. You have no idea why someone is doing what they are doing or how they are doing it. Whatever you see, is all your perception and interpretation. It will always differ from one person to the other.

The other important thing is that you should not judge yourself. So what if you lose balance when doing that pose, or you accidentally trip and fall? The one thing you should remember is that someone has done something silly and embarrassing before and no one judges you. So, why are you too hard on yourself?

Practice on a full stomach

Just as we have mentioned this point before, it is important that you do not have a big meal right before yoga class. If you are attending a class, you can have a meal 2-3 hours before yoga practice. This will not only ensure that you are energized for the class, but also will keep you from feeling like throwing up during sessions.

If you feel as though you are starving and cannot wait until the end of the class, you can grab something light to keep you going. You can have a light snack like a banana, nuts, yogurt or a smoothie.

Bring your phone

One of the common sources of distractions during practice is a phone ringing, beeping or texts coming in. When you get into your yoga class, ensure that you completely unplug. You can either mute it or switch it off and leave it back in your locker room to avoid the temptation of turning it on to check an email or call home etc. You are aware of how distracting receiving a phone call is in class, and I expect that you know how disrespectful it is, not just the class, but also to your instructor.

Self-compare to others

The truth is, at some point, there will always be someone more flexible than us, thinner, lighter, fashionable, beautiful, sharper, among other things. This should not bother you one bit. We all start from somewhere, and your body is different from that of your neighbor and so are other people.

Rather than comparing yourself to others, take snapshots of your journey during practice. When you do this, you will start to see the difference and the progress you are making. You will appreciate that you too deserve a pat on your back for the great work done.

Use hand cream before class

When I first took yoga classes, I worked in a retail food shop, and I have to be in gloves whenever I am working. Gloves often leave a certain smell and powder on the hands that you have to ensure that you wash your hands soon after disposing of them. So, often I would apply hand cream after washing my hands and heading for yoga classes.

I very quickly realized that this was a bad idea! This is because the hand cream tends to make the hands moist and you tend to slide a lot on the mat. I kept wiping hands on my pants over and over, and this was more distracting than anything else.

Yes, you may not be working in a retail food shop as I did in my earlier years, but applying the cream on your hands can be a terrible mistake.

CHAPTER EIGHT

FAQs for Yoga Beginners

1. Which form of yoga should I practice?

There are so many forms of yoga that we have discussed above. Choosing the right form of yoga to practice often depends on a wide range of factors like; age, level of yoga you are at, your fitness goals among others. Other yoga is slow paced while others are fast-paced. The other will be restorative while others are meditative.

The most important thing is for you to experiment with different forms to appreciate how different each one is until you get one that suits you and gives you exactly what you are looking for if not more!

2. How do I identify the best yoga instructor?

As mentioned earlier, identifying a good instructor is very important. This is often the case if you are a beginner. All you have to do is ask around or attend a couple of introductory sessions at several yoga studios to find the one that you connect with. Also, ensure that the teacher you are working with is not only trained but also registered with a reputable institution.

Also, look out for someone that speaks to you, offers clear instructions and makes it their priority to keep you safe during class. They should be someone that makes you feel comfortable and welcome in their class.

3. Is it possible to learn yoga online?

Yes, it is possible to learn yoga online. There are so many online resources that you can follow at the comfort of your home. However, it is critical that if you are a beginner, you should find a good yoga instructor that will help you avoid as many mistakes as you possibly can to keep safe. You can do it at home during your free time to master a couple of poses.

4. Do I need to be flexible to be in a yoga class?

It is a class because you are learning. So, to answer this question; No! If you are flexible while starting yoga, that is great. However, if you are not flexible, yoga is what you need to gain that flexibility and balance.

5. If I am overweight, can I still practice yoga?

Yes, yoga is for everyone irrespective of your body weight, shape, race, and status. If you are overweight, your instructor will help you by making modifications on the poses to help accommodate your body size and shape so that you can benefit from practice.

6. Can I lose weight with yoga?

Indeed, yoga can help you shed off extra pounds. Employing a couple of gentle postures together with mindful breathing goes a long way in ensuring that your body gets rid of toxins, cleanses the body and lowers the risk of developing stress and anxiety related disorders.

One of the biggest culprits when it comes to weight gain is stress. Yoga can lower stress levels and hence, provide gentle exercises that will strengthen the body and tone the muscles.

7. How many times in a week do I have to practice?

It is advisable that you practice at least once a day; however short the session might be. It is hugely beneficial when you just get out of bed in the morning. You can sign up for yoga so that you stay focused and energized throughout the day. However, one thing that you should remember is you can do yoga everywhere. You can practice it in the living room and will equally be the same as what you do in class.

8. Is yoga strenuous?

It could be. This is especially the case for modern yoga classes. Some of the yoga poses may be gentle and relaxing, while others may be vigorous and strenuous. If you are a beginner, it is crucial that you start with basic yoga poses that are designed for people who are new to yoga.

Once you have mastered your yoga poses and achieved a certain level of flexibility and confidence, you can start branching out. This allows you to find a yoga style that sits well with your body shape and fitness goals.

9. Will I have muscle cramps and sores after class?

Well, if you are a beginner, sometimes you may experience muscle cramps during the first few weeks of starting yoga. This may be because there is a combination of muscles that are used when practicing and because they were not used to this before, they are trying to adjust.

The soreness is normal, it's actually a great initial sign. However, if you keep at it, the soreness begins to fade away. If the muscle cramps become worse and intolerable, you can reduce the number of sessions you have in a week or the length of time you practice per session just until your body eases in well.

10. How many beginner sessions should I attend to move to the next level?

This is one of the most common questions among beginners. It indicates how mindful they are at approaching yoga practice, something great. For me, taking about 8-10 beginner sessions may be enough for you to start taking on challenging poses. However, one thing that you have to realize is that this also depends on your body.

If you feel that the poses you are doing are manageable and not challenging, then you need to move on. However, if you still find it difficult to balance and are struggling with flexibility, you need to work on that before you can proceed to the next level. Ensure that you keep an open mind, rest when you need to and do your best.

Just remember, I revisit beginner classes on occasions because it's a great way to really focus on your technique and positions. Sometimes, correcting your technique is more important and impactful on your body compared to undergoing more complex and strenuous poses.

11. Should I use props during yoga classes?

Indeed, there are times when you need props to offer you support during practice. However, using these items such as prop, straps, and blankets will not enhance your practice but are important when you are a beginner.

You can use these items to get the support you need when you need that extra balance. One thing that you have to remember is that using props has nothing to do with experience. Regardless of how long you have been practicing yoga, you may need props to help you do one thing or another.

12. How long do I need to practice before I can start to see changes?

When you are a beginner, it is normal to want to see changes immediately. Well, in as much as this is a good attitude, the truth is that you may not see the changes that soon. You have to keep practicing yoga as much as you can, and soon you start seeing the difference.

When you start feeling like the muscles are getting sore, it means that you are gaining certain strength, flexibility, and improved well-being. You will soon experience changes in your weight. All you have to do is stick to the routine and ensure that you challenge yourself every day. Also, be aware of positive changes when they start happening. These changes may include improved sleep patterns, increased focus, and feelings of relaxation. All these are rewarding feelings and changes that we all are working towards achieving.

Conclusion

Indeed, yoga is a lifestyle and not a religion, cult or belief. It is at the root of yoga that you find self-inquiry and an understanding of your body. Everything that you do through yoga \will bring you a sense of purpose so that you stay encouraged to work towards connecting to your body. It is what contributes significantly to giving our lives more meaning in a way.

One of the things that you have to remember at all times is that yoga helps you understand the balance of effort, constant focus, and sensitivity in your daily activities. It will help you relieve stress and achieve relaxation. When you start experiencing relaxation, you start to feel a deep reward from within. You start to feel that nothing can stand in the way of your dreams even when faced with extremely challenging situations. You get to do those hard poses effortlessly with a calm mind and steady breathing.

It is through yoga that you get a deeper sense of self-understanding. It is what gives you that strong physical, emotional and spiritual wellbeing. It is indeed, much more than a simple physical experience. Yoga digs deeper into uncovering the reality of who you are. You begin to let go of the past so that you can embrace what lies in your future. You feel happier, more connected and content with your life and the people around you.

I hope that this book helps you see all this and more about yoga. If you eventually begin your first class, know that we wish you the very best and believe that you are going to have a fruitful, purposeful and more impactful lifestyle than you have ever dreamed possible.

So, what is it going to be for you today? Are you ready to take a leap of faith and sign up for a yoga class in your neighborhood? Don't wait too long because your time is now! All that fitness, self-understanding, physical, emotional and spiritual wellbeing is waiting for you.